Contents

Mechanical Soft Diet

The mechanical soft diet can be used if you are having trouble chewing and/or swallowing. Eating soft foods promotes healing and helps prevent choking or breathing in food particles or liquids (aspiration). "Mechanical" refers to making food softer, smaller, and easier to eat through the use of kitchen implements like blenders, food processors, and grinders.

Why a Mechanical Soft Diet May Be Recommended

Dysphagia can cause a variety of serious problems. In addition to choking, you could aspirate food or liquids into your lungs, putting you at risk for pneumonia or chest congestion. Also, if you are unable to swallow food or drink, you are at risk for weight loss, malnutrition and dehydration.

You can have trouble swallowing for a variety of reasons. You may be missing teeth or have poorly fitting dentures, making it difficult to chew food properly. You may be recovering from mouth or neck surgery. Or you may have a medical condition or injury, such as:

- Neurological disorder, including multiple sclerosis, muscular dystrophy, and Parkinson's disease

- Stroke

- Brain or spinal cord injury

- Alzheimer's disease

- Cancer of the throat or neck

- Cancer treatment effects, such as from radiation to the head, neck or throat

- Problems with the esophagus, such as narrowing, tumors or tissue damage due to GERD (gastroesophageal reflux disease)

- Conditions that cause reduced saliva, such as Sjogren syndrome

- Pharyngoesophageal diverticulum, or Zenker's diverticulum, a condition in which food particles are collected in a pouch in the throat

If you have dysphagia for these or any other reason, your doctor is likely to put you on a special diet to make it easier for you to eat or drink.

Benefits

The soft mechanical diet helps you get balanced nutrition despite not being able to chew or swallow easily and/or without discomfort.

Your doctor may suggest the diet if you have a swallowing disorder (dysphagia); are experiencing a sore throat, head, and/or neck after receiving radiation therapy; or have dental pain from adjusting to dentures or braces.

You may also need to be on a mechanical soft diet while recovering from an illness or surgery involving your digestive tract, as soft foods tend to be easier on your system.

The mechanical soft diet can also be used as a "bridge" to help you transition back to your regular diet after being on a liquid diet.

How It Works

The main goal of the mechanical soft diet is avoiding foods that require a lot of chewing, such as tough meat, raw veggies, bread with a thick crust, nuts, seeds, and hard or crunchy snacks.

Some foods, such as pudding, are safe for a mechanical soft diet as is. Other foods, like vegetables, require a little more work. You can still eat most foods on a mechanical soft diet as long as they have safe consistency.

Your choice of food is limited by texture more than ingredients, so it's possible to eat a well-balanced, varied, and flavorful diet—especially with help from the right tools.

Duration

A mechanical soft diet is usually only necessary for a short period of time, such as while you're recovering from an illness, injury, or surgery.

If a mechanical soft diet is necessary for longer—for example, if you have lost most of your teeth or have suffered a severe jaw injury—you will need to work closely with your healthcare team to ensure you stay nourished and hydrated. You may also find it helpful to work with a registered dietitian or nutritionist who can guide you through the process of creating a nutritious meal plan.

What to Eat

If a particular food requires a lot of chewing, you can assume it's not allowed on a mechanical soft diet—at least, not in its original form.

All liquids are allowed on a mechanical soft diet, assuming they do not contain nuts and seeds, tapioca pearls or boba, chunks of fruit, or pieces of candy.

Foods To eat

- Cooked vegetables (mashed and skinned)

- Canned fruit

- Applesauce

- Stewed fruit (remove skin, pits, or seeds)

- Avocado

- Farina

- Oatmeal

- Cereal with milk

- White bread, crackers (softened with milk)

- Cooked white rice or pasta

- Yogurt

- Soft cheese, cottage cheese, cream cheese

- Clear broth, creamed soups

- Baked, poached, or broiled fish

- Ground or thinly-shaved meat (turkey, chicken, beef, pork)

- Soft-cooked eggs, egg salad

- Tuna, chicken

- Silken tofu

- Hummus

- Ice cream, pudding, custard (no nuts)

- Soft cakes or cookies (no nuts, candy, raisins)

- Condiments, gravy, sauces, spices

- Butter, vegetable/cooking oils, margarine

Foods To Avoid

- Hard cheese, cheese with nuts or seeds

- Shellfish and "meaty" fish (e.g., haddock, halibut)

- Hot dogs, sausage

- Fried meat or fish

- Nuts and seeds

- Crunchy nut butters

- Raw vegetables

- Whole fruit with skin, pits, or seeds

- Dried fruit

- Whole olives

- Coconut

- Bread, muffins, cakes, or cookies with seeds, nuts, or dried fruit

- Crunchy bread (rye, pumpernickel, sourdough)

- Kasha buckwheat or wild rice

- Shredded wheat

- Granola

- French fries, hash browns

- Toast

- Crackers, melba toast, croutons

- Chips, popcorn, pretzels, crunchy cookies

- Granola bars

- Pie crust

- Chewy or hard candy

- Jams/jelly with seeds

Fruits and vegetables: Fruits and vegetables can be peeled, cooked, mashed or strained, and easily blended to make them safe for a mechanical soft diet. Some produce, like avocado, is ready to eat as-is. Mash or purée other fruits and veggies, just remember to remove any seeds first.

Prepackaged frozen produce is convenient and often softer right out of the package.

Grains: Avoid dry, hard cereals, as well as granola with nuts, seeds, dried fruit, or candy.

Hot cereals like farina, oatmeal, and grits work well for a mechanical soft diet as long as you don't add nuts, berries, or other toppings. Try tossing in mushy fruit like bananas instead.

Soft bread can be used to make sandwiches with egg, chicken, or tuna salad. Avoid toasting bread or choosing varieties with hard, crispy crusts, such as sourdough.

Dairy: Dairy products like yogurt, soft cheese, and cottage cheese are already suitable for a mechanical soft diet without any additional prep.

Protein: Meat is allowed on a mechanical soft diet with special prep. Remove fat or gristle and cook the meat until tender. Use gravy and sauce to moisten the meat and help prevent it from becoming tough. Ground meat can also be puréed. Soften canned tuna with mayonnaise or water.

Soft-cooked, poached, or scrambled eggs, egg whites, and egg substitutes are also a good choice for a mechanical soft diet.

If you don't eat animal products, plant-based protein sources like smooth nut butter, mashed up beans, and silken tofu are all approved.[1]

Desserts: Soft cakes, cookies, and custards are allowed as long as they don't have any pieces of candy, nuts, or seeds in them. Ice cream, sorbet, and other frozen treats are easy to swallow and can be soothing to a sore throat or mouth.

Avoid any sticky, chewy, or crunchy candies like caramels, licorice, and lollipops.

Beverages: All liquids are allowed and are necessary for staying hydrated while you're on a mechanical soft diet. If you're making shakes, smoothies, or blended drinks, just make sure there aren't any large pieces of fruit, nuts, or other solids.

Recommended Timing

In general, you should be able to follow your regular schedule for eating. However, if you are eating fewer calories, you may need to eat more often to ensure you are getting enough nutrition each day.

Cooking Tips

Kitchen appliances and gadgets such as blenders and food processors can make the task of preparing soft foods much easier, but they certainly aren't required.

A knife is sufficient for chopping food into smaller pieces. Once cut, many foods can be softened up in the oven, on the stove, or in the microwave. A regular fork is often sufficient for mashing. Adding gravy, sauce, oils, butter, or a little water can help your efforts.

If you need to add nutrition or calories, nutrition powders, yeasts, and supplements can be tossed into milkshakes and smoothies, sprinkled on oats or yogurt, or mixed into a warm beverage.

Once you find some meals you like and that work for the mechanical soft diet, prepare larger batches and freeze them.

For beverages, you can usually stick to your preference for how they're served. Avoid any extreme temperatures, as well as ice with sharp edges.

Modifications

If you have other medical conditions, your doctor may suggest additional restrictions to a basic mechanical soft diet to help control your symptoms.

For example, if you have gastroesophageal reflux disease (GERD) or a dental problem, you will likely need to avoid spicy or acidic foods and drinks, which can cause or worsen irritation.[1]

If you follow a special diet, such as gluten-free, vegan, vegetarian, or low-FODMAP, you can easily incorporate approved foods into a mechanical soft diet. However, if you need to add liquid nutritional supplements, you will want to carefully check the list of ingredients for allergens.

Considerations

Components of a mechanical soft diet can be adjusted to match your appetite, tastes, and nutritional needs. While flexible in these regards, there are some considerations to keep in mind.

General Nutrition

Just as you would with your regular diet, you'll want to be sure to get a good mix of protein, fat, carbohydrates, and fiber, as well as essential vitamins and minerals. Of course, when you're feeling sick or in pain, this can be challenging. You may also have a hard time drinking enough fluids to prevent dehydration.

If you need to be on a mechanical soft diet for more than a few days, check with your healthcare team to ensure that your body is getting what it needs.

Sustainability and Practicality

Making foods work for a mechanical soft diet can require a bit of work. If you know you will need to be on the diet to recover from a planned procedure, you will have some time to plan ahead. This might include stocking up on healthy foods that are easy to chew as well as chopping, cooking, and softening fruits, veggies, and meats.

If you are too sick to prepare food or are on a mechanical soft diet unexpectedly, look for foods and beverages that require little preparation. If you have others who can help with food prep, make sure they have the guidelines for a mechanical soft diet handy.

Safety

A mechanical soft diet should be easy enough to consume that the risk of pain and choking is very low. However, these things are possible if you're not careful about food preparation—for example, meat is cut just a tad too large or a vegetable isn't steamed enough.

Be mindful in the kitchen and with what you are served. You can also consider asking a loved one to assess the consistency of something before you take a bite.

Cost

Beyond your typical grocery bill, other costs you may want to consider are the tools and appliances that could make preparing food for a mechanical soft diet easier.

For example, a basic blender or mini food chopper can be purchased for around $20. Food processors are typically more expensive (closer to $50). You may also want to invest in a good, sharp knife for chopping, which can cost as low as $20 or much more.

Energy and General Health

When you're primarily eating soft foods and liquids, it can be difficult to figure out how many calories you're getting. If you feel like you aren't eating enough to keep your strength up or you notice you're losing weight, talk to your doctor.

Depending on what you include in a soft mechanical diet, you may not be able to get all the vitamins and minerals you need. If you notice you are very tired, have bleeding gums, are not thinking clearly, or have other symptoms that concern you, make sure you let your doctor know. You may have a deficiency in a certain nutrient that's causing your symptoms.

Mechanical Soft Diet vs. Other Diets

The mechanical soft diet is similar to several other diets used to treat pain and other symptoms associated with digestive disorders. These diets may also be used to help patients prepare or recover from surgery.

However, these diets are generally much more restrictive because they limit food groups based on attributes other than consistency, such as fiber or fat content.

Soft (Puréed) Diet

The main difference between the two diets is that the mechanical soft diet is focused on reducing the amount of chewing necessary, while a soft diet is not.[1]

A soft diet is usually prescribed for people who are recovering from bowel surgery or have digestive disorders. You may also need to be on a soft diet to prepare for a procedure or test such as endoscopy or colonoscopy.

Liquid Diet

A full liquid diet may be necessary if you can't eat or digest any solid food at all. People with medical emergencies like bowel obstruction may be limited to a liquid-only diet while they recover or if they need an operation.

When preparing for surgery, you may be told you can only have clear liquids. If you're already eating a mechanical soft diet, many of the approved foods can be made suitable for a liquid diet if you thin them out with water.

Mechanical Soft Diet (Level 1 to 3)

Mechanical soft diets are less restrictive than a soft food diet. Foods that aren't normally soft can be eaten, once you puree, blend, chop, whip or grind them using blenders, food processors, or other devices. Mechanical diets also do not restrict fat, fiber, spices and seasonings, which soft diets often exclude.

The National Dysphagia Diet Guidelines list three mechanical soft food diet plans, depending on a person's chewing and swallowing abilities. However, advice regarding specific foods may vary depending on each person's individual comfort level. A doctor or registered dietitian may need to tailor a mechanical soft foods diet plan for each patient.

Here are the general guidelines:

• Level 1: Foods are pureed, with consistent and uniform textures—no surprise chunks. They are easy to swallow without any chewing required. Foods for this level include pudding, custard, yogurt, oatmeal, pureed fruits and pureed meats.

• Level 2: Foods are moist, with soft texture for easy swallowing. These can include small bites (for example, pieces of meat are ground or cut so that pieces are no bigger than a quarter of an inch). Some mixed textures are allowed, such as in casseroles. Level 1 foods can be given, plus such foods as soft pancakes moistened with syrup, soft canned fruits, soft meats like fish, moist macaroni, and scrambled eggs.

- Level 3: Food at this stage is much closer to normal, but should still be moist and bite-size. It also excludes foods that are very hard, sticky, crunchy or overly dry. Mechanical soft food diet foods to avoid at this level include dry bread, toast, crackers, coarse cereal like shredded wheat, foods with nuts, fruits that are hard to chew (such as apples), seeds, chunky peanut butter, and meats that are tough and dry.

Liquids as Part of a Mechanical Soft Food Diet Plan

Depending on how severe a person's dysphagia, liquids may have to be thickened with thickening agents like cornstarch or gelatin. (Pre-thickened liquids are available commercially.) If you or someone you care for is on a mechanical soft food diet, your healthcare provider may determine the safe level of beverage thickness you can tolerate.

Liquid consistency levels include:

• "Pudding thick" or "spoon thick." This requires drinks to be thickened to such a degree that they require eating with a spoon.

• "Honey thick." Drinks must be prepared so they are the consistency of honey. They can't be ingested with a straw.

• "Nectar thick." Drinks are thickened to nectar or maple-syrup consistency.

• Thin liquids. These are drinks at normal consistency.

Anything that melts at room temperature is treated as a liquid. That means ice cream, popsicles or sherbet should not be served to someone with dysphagia unless they are able to ingest them at their melted consistency.

A mechanical soft food diet can be a lifelong diet or may be only temporary, depending on the reason for dysphagia. For example, many stroke patients may need to be on this diet at first, but as brain inflammation recedes, they may be able to return to a normal diet. Therapy with a speech-language pathologist may help some people improve their ability to swallow.

Planning Your Meals

Changing your eating habits can be hard. It's best to plan ahead for meals. This can help make sure you have enough of the right foods to eat at mealtimes. Here are some questions to think about when planning your meals:

• Where will you be eating? (At home, a restaurant, work, someone else's house)

• If you're eating at a restaurant, can you call ahead and request special meals?

• Will you have a kitchen and refrigerator available? Can you boil water? Can you microwave? Can you use a blender or food processor?

• Can you carry a thermos with food already prepared and ready to eat?

Eating at home with family and friends

Most foods can be changed to meet your needs. For example, a portion of soup can be put aside, then strained or blended.

Many main dishes, such as noodles, stews, and casseroles, can be put into a blender with some liquid. You can use milk, gravy, tomato sauce, broth, juice, or water. Add liquid until the food is the right consistency.

Kitchen items to help prepare foods

Here are some items that you may find helpful to prepare your foods at home:

Blender: You can use a blender for all types of foods including meats, vegetables and fruits, but you may have to add liquid to make the food the right texture. Blenders are great for soups and shakes. However, they're not always the best to use for making 1 portion.

The Magic Bullet® and Nutribullet®These are small blenders that don't take up a lot of space. The Vitamix® and Ninja® are other powerful blenders that can purée a variety of foods.

Hand-held blender: You can use a hand-held blender to quickly purée your favorite soups right in the pot. It can also be used to soften well-cooked foods in a small bowl for 1 or 2 portions.

Food processor: Food processors are useful for shredding, slicing, chopping, or blending foods. It comes in different sizes. If you often prepare just 1 portion of food, buy a small processor.

Household mesh strainer or sieve: You can use this to strain fruits and vegetables, but not meats. They are inexpensive, good to make 1 portion, and don't need electricity. However, this method can be slow.

Baby-food grinder: This item can often be found in stores that sell baby clothes or furniture. They are good for all foods and require no liquid. The small ones are ideal for grinding 1 portion of food. They can be hand or battery-operated.

However, when using a baby-food grinder, food may not come out as smooth as some people may need. Ask your dietitian, doctor, or speech or swallowing therapist if it's right for you.

Eating Out

Eat at restaurants that offer a variety of foods and that will cater to people on special diets. Many places will purée or prepare foods for your needs. Call ahead and speak to a manager or chef. You may be surprised at how helpful they will be. You may also want to order sides of broth, gravy, or milk to moisten your foods.

Here are some ideas of things you can order. Some of these may need to be mashed or blended for the puréed diet:

Breakfast

• Fruit and vegetable juices

• Fruits

• Hot cereal

- Cold cereal softened in milk (for mechanical soft diets)

- Scrambled eggs or chopped, hard-boiled eggs for mechanical soft diets

- Soft breads, such as muffins and pancakes, soaked in liquid to soften them for mechanical soft diets

- Coffee, tea, or hot chocolate

Lunch and dinner

- Fruit and vegetable juices

- Soups, which can be easily blended or strained in the restaurant. Egg drop soup is a good source of protein

Main dishes

- Ground meat products, such as hamburger patties, meatloaf, and meatballs

- Soft, flaky fish (such as fillet of sole, flounder, or tilapia) steamed, baked, or broiled

- Noodles and macaroni dishes, blended for puréed diets

- Soufflés

- Cottage cheese and soft fruit platters

- Sandwiches, such as tuna or egg salad on soft bread

Vegetables

- Baked or mashed potatoes

- Any soft cooked vegetables, such as cooked carrots

- Creamed spinach

- Vegetable soufflé

- Guacamole (some may be spicy)

- Hummus

Desserts

- Ice cream or frozen yogurt

- Gelatin desserts

- Milkshakes

- Mousse

- Puddings and custards

- Applesauce or other soft fruits

- Fruit sorbets

It's also possible to eat away from home, such as at work or at a friend's house. Here are some tips for taking food with you while you're away from home:

• Bring a food grinder or small food processor. If electricity is needed, make sure it's available where you're going.

• Buy a thermos. Make soup or hot cereal and carry it with you.

• Ask if there is a microwave where you're going. You can make food at home and freeze it in portion-sized, microwave-safe containers or Zip-Loc® bags. Bring the food with you in an insulated pack and heat it when you want to eat.

• Freeze soups or puréed foods in ice cube trays. Cover the tray with foil or plastic wrap to prevent freezer burn. When you're hungry, use 2 or 3 cubes for a small meal or snack, or more cubes for a larger meal.

• Fruit ices

Your Caloric Needs

Your caloric needs are the number of calories you need every day to maintain your weight. You get calories from food and drinks. Eating the number of calories your body needs can help you maintain your weight.

You can adjust the amount of calories you eat in order to reach your weight goal:

• If you need to gain weight, you can increase the number of calories you eat or drink.

• If you need to lose weight, you can decrease the number of calories you eat or drink.

Each person has needs a different number of calories. This is based on:

• Age

• Sex

• Height and weight

• Level of physical activity

Generally, people who are older or less active need fewer calories. Your doctor and dietitian can help you find out how many calories you need every day

The easiest way to check if you're eating enough is to weigh yourself. Try to weigh yourself twice a week and write down how much you weigh.

This will help you keep track of your weight loss or gain.

Tips for adding more calories to your diet

If you need to eat more calories, here are some easy tips:

• Eat small meals 6 to 8 times a day instead of 3 main meals.

• Add 2 to 4 tablespoons of canned coconut milk or cream to smoothies, shakes, cereals, or yogurts for extra calories. You can also add it to rice or diced chicken for extra calories, flavor, and moisture.

• Choose creamy soups rather than soups with clear broths.

• Have puddings and custards rather than gelatin desserts, such as Jell-O®.

• Add sauces, gravies, or extra vegetable oil to your meals.

• Drink apricot, pear, or peach fruit nectars. They are less acidic than other nectars.

• Drink fruit shakes or fruit smoothies made with yogurt or ice cream.

• Make ice cubes from milk or fruit nectar. Use these high-calorie ice cubes in smoothies or to keep your shakes cold. As they melt, they will add calories to your beverages.

• Drink high-calorie drinks, such as milkshakes, soy milkshakes, or pasteurized eggnog.

• Drink a liquid nutritional supplement, such as Ensure or Boost, instead of milk to make a nutritious, high-calorie milkshake.

• Add honey to smoothies, tea, yogurt, hot cereals, shakes, or ice cream.

• If you aren't on a low-fat diet, add sour cream, half and half, heavy cream, or whole milk to your foods. You can add it to mashed potatoes, sauces, gravies, cereals, soups, and casseroles.

• Add mayonnaise to your eggs, chicken, tuna, pasta, or potatoes to make a smooth, moist salad.

• Add avocado to dishes or smoothies.

• Add nut butters, such as peanut butter, to shakes and smoothies.

Tips for adding more protein to your diet

If you need to increase the amount of protein in your diet, here are some easy tips:

• Add tofu to cooked vegetables, soups, smoothies, or in place of chicken or meat if you're having difficulty eating animal proteins.

• Add cooked eggs to your soups, broths, and cooked vegetables. Purée the cooked eggs, if needed.

• Use plain Greek yogurt in smoothies, cream sauces, or wherever you would use sour cream.

• Use a plain protein powder, such as a whey protein powder, in liquids and shakes.

- Add cheese (shredded or grated) to your soups, cooked eggs, vegetables, and starches.

For example, adding full-fat ricotta cheese can moisten a dish and add calories and protein. Add cottage cheese to smoothies, purées, or canned fruits.

- Use fortified milk (see recipe in the "Recipes" section) rather than regular milk to double the amount of protein in it. Use this milk in shakes, hot cereals, mashed potatoes, hot chocolate, or with instant puddings to create a high-protein, high-calorie dessert. You can also add non-fat dried milk powder alone to purées and smoothies to add more calories and protein.

• Grind some nuts with a coffee grinder and add to them to your smoothies, hot cereals, puddings, or yogurts.

Liquid nutritional supplements

If you can't make your own shakes, there are many nutritional supplements that you can buy. Some are high calorie, ready-prepared drinks that have vitamins and minerals added to them. Others are powders that you can mix into other foods or drinks. Most are also lactose-free, which means that you can have them even if you're lactose intolerant

Sample menu for a mechanical soft diet

Here are some examples of meals you can have when you're on a mechanical soft diet. If you need help planning your meals, call the

Department of Food and Nutrition to speak with a dietitian.

Mechanical Soft Diet Meal Plan

Breakfast

- Soft, diced peaches

- Cereal softened in milk

- Diced, soft pancakes with syrup and butter

- Scrambled eggs

- A soft butter roll cut into small pieces

Mid-morning

- Yogurt

Lunch

- Vegetable barley soup

* Chicken salad or egg salad

* Diced, well-cooked spinach

* Canned fruit cocktail

Mid-afternoon snack

* Ensure plus

Dinner

* Soup

* Baked fish filet (boneless) with sauce

* Diced, soft potatoes

* Diced, well-cooked broccoli with olive oil or butter

* Canned, diced pears

Evening Snack

* Rice Pudding

MECHANICAL SOFT DIET RECIPES

Trying mechanical soft-friendly recipes is a great way to explore new flavors and find new favorite dishes while looking after your health. In this part are nourishing mechanical soft diet recipes for you to enjoy.

Peanut butter and banana Sandwich

Preparation time

5 minutes

Ingredients:

- 4 tablespoons of peanut butter

- 1 banana, sliced

- 4 slices of soft bread

Instructions:

1. Spread 2 tablespoons of peanut butter on each of two slices of bread.

2. Place half of the banana slices on each of the two slices of bread on top of the peanut butter.

3. Place the other slice of bread on top of each sandwich.

4. Cut eat sandwich in half and serve.

Easy Chicken and dumplings

Preparation time

20 minutes

Ingredients

- 2 cans mixed vegetables

- 3 cans chicken broth

- 3 cups cubed cooked chicken breast

- 1/8 teaspoon garlic powder

- 1/8 teaspoon pepper

- 1-2/3 cups biscuit/baking mix

- 2/3 cup milk

Instructions:

1. In a large pot, stir in the broth, chicken, garlic powder, and pepper.

2. Bring to a boil, then reduce heat to low/simmer.

3. Drain canned mixed vegetables and gently stir into the mixture.

4. For dumplings, combine biscuit mix and milk.

5. Drop tablespoonfuls into simmering broth mixture.

6. Cover and simmer for 10-15 minutes.

7. A toothpick can be inserted into dumplings and removed clean when dumplings are cooked.

Slow Cooker Pot Roast

Preparation time

9 hours 10 minutes

Ingredients:

- 2 cans condensed cream of mushroom soup

- 1 package dry onion soup mix

- 1 1/2 cups beef broth

- 5-6 pounds of pot roast

- 1 package of baby carrots

- 1/2 pound of pearl onions

Instructions

1. Place pot roast in slow cooker, and pour carrots and onions on top.

2. In a mixing bowl, mix cream of mushroom soup, dry onion soup mix and beef broth.

3. Pour soup mixture over carrots, onions, and pot roast.

4. Cook on Low setting for 9 hours, or until roast, carrots, and onions are very soft and tender, so that the meat falls apart easily.

Easy Meatloaf

Preparation time

1 hour 10 minutes

Ingredients:

- 1 1/2 pounds ground beef

- 2 eggs

- 1/2 cup each: onion and green bell pepper, finely chopped or pureed

- 3/4 cup milk

- 1 cup dried bread crumbs

- 1/8 teaspoon each salt, pepper, and garlic powder

- 2 tablespoons each: sugar and molasses

- 2 tablespoons yellow mustard

- 1/3 cup ketchup

Instructions:

1. Preheat oven to 350 degrees.

2. In a large mixing bowl, combine the beef, egg, onion, milk and bread crumbs. Season with salt, pepper, and garlic powder.

3. Spoon mixture into a greased 5x9 inch loaf pan, or form into a loaf and place in a lightly greased baking dish.

4. In a separate small bowl, combine the sugar, molasses, mustard and ketchup.

5. Mix well and pour over the meatloaf.

6. Bake at 350 degrees for 1 hour.

Chicken Rockefeller Pasta

Prepartion time

15 minutes

Ingredients:

- 1 can (10-3/4 ounces) condensed cream of chicken soup

- 1 cup milk

- 3/4 cup grated Cheddar cheese

- 1/8 teaspoon each pepper and garlic powder

- 1 package of wide egg noodles

- 2 large cans of cooked chicken

- 1 can of spinach, drained

Instructions:

1. Prepare the noodles by the package instructions.

2. Meanwhile, in a large saucepan, combine the soup, milk, cheddar cheese, pepper, and garlic.

3. After the cheese has melted and the mixture is smooth, stir in the chicken and the spinach.

4. After the noodles are cooked and drained, spoon noodles onto a plate and spoon sauce on top of the noodles.

Chicken and Broccoli Pasta

Prepartion time

15 minutes

Ingredients:

- 1 can (10-3/4 ounces) condensed cream of chicken soup

- 1 cup milk

- 1/2 cup grated Parmesan cheese

- 1/8 teaspoon each pepper and garlic powder

- 1 package of wide egg noodles

- 2 large cans of cooked chicken

- 1 bag of microwave steam broccoli

Instructions:

1. Prepare the noodles by the package instructions.

2. Prepare the broccoli in the microwave per package instructions, making sure it is cooked well enough that it is soft.

3. Meanwhile, in a large saucepan, combine the soup, milk, Parmesan cheese, pepper, and garlic powder.

4. After the cheese has melted and the mixture is smooth, stir in the chicken and the broccoli.

5. After the noodles are cooked and drained, stir in the noodles and serve.

Chicken, Peas and Carrot Pasta

Prepartion time

15 minutes

Ingredients:

- 1 can (10-3/4 ounces) condensed cream of chicken soup

- 1 cup milk

- 1/2 cup grated Parmesan cheese

- 1/8 teaspoon each pepper and garlic powder

- 1 package of wide egg noodles

- 2 large cans of cooked chicken

- 1 can of peas and carrots

Instructions:

1. Prepare the noodles by the package instructions.

2. Meanwhile, in a large saucepan, combine the soup, milk, Parmesan cheese, pepper, and garlic.

3. After the cheese has melted and the mixture is smooth, stir in the chicken and the peas and carrots.

4. After the noodles are cooked and drained, stir in the noodles and serve.

Chicken and Noodles

Prepartion time

15 minutes

Ingredients:

- 1 can (10-3/4 ounces) condensed cream of chicken soup

- 1 cup milk

- 1/2 cup grated Parmesan cheese

- 1/8 teaspoon pepper

- 1 package of wide egg noodles

- 2 large cans of cooked chicken

Instructions:

1. Prepare the noodles by the package instructions.

2. Meanwhile, in a large saucepan, combine the soup, milk, Parmesan cheese and pepper.

3. After the cheese has melted and the mixture is smooth, stir in the chicken.

4. After the noodles are cooked and drained, stir in the noodles and serve.

Tortellini pasta Alfredo

Prepartion time

25 minutes

Ingredients:

- 1 package frozen cheese tortellini

- 1 cup heavy whipping cream

- 1/8 teaspoon garlic powder

- 1/2 cup butter slices

- 1 cup shredded Parmesan cheese

Instructions:

1. Begin to boil tortellini according to package directions.

2. While tortellini is cooking, combine cream, butter slices, and garlic powder into a small saucepan.

3. Cook, uncovered, over medium-low heat until heated but not boiling. Turn off heat.

4. Stir in Parmesan cheese until melted and smooth.

5. Drain pasta and put drained tortellini pasta in a large serving bowl.

6. Pour Alfredo sauce over pasta.

7. Gently toss to coat pasta.

Quick Cherry Tarts

Prepartion time

15 minutes

Ingredients:

• 1 can cherry pie filling (21 oz.)

• 6 single-serve graham cracker crusts

• 1 package of whipped cream topping, thawed

Optional:

- Chocolate Syrup

Instructions:

1. Spoon pie filling into the crusts, dividing equally between the crusts.

2. Top with whipped cream topping.

3. Drizzle with chocolate syrup if desired.

Baked Dill Salmon

Preparation time

30 minutes

Ingredients

- 1 large salmon fillet (2 pounds)

- 2 tablespoons butter, softened

- 2 tablespoons mayonnaise

- 2 tablespoons lemon juice

- 1/2 teaspoon pepper

- 1/2 teaspoon dried dill

Instructions:

1. Pat salmon dry. Grease 13 x 9" baking dish.

2. Place salmon in baking dish.

3. Combine remaining ingredients and spread over salmon.

4. Bake, uncovered, at 425° for 20-25 minutes or until salmon flakes easily with a fork.

5. Serve with mashed potatoes and/or well cooked, soft vegetables.

Egg and Olive Salad sandwich

Prepartion time

10 minutes

Ingredients:

- 2 boiled, peeled eggs, finely chopped

- 1/4 cup of chopped green olives with pimentos

- 1 Tablespoon of Mayonnaise

- 4 slices of soft bread

Instructions:

1. Mix the eggs, olives, and mayonnaise together.

2. Spread half of the mixture on each of two slices of bread.

3. Place the other slice of bread on top of each sandwich.

4. Makes two full sandwiches, or three if you prefer less filling for each sandwich.

Savoury Bread Pudding with Lots of Veg

Prepartion time

45 minutes

Ingredients

- oil or oil spray, for greasing your dish

- 150 g (approximately) day-old bread, crusts removed & cut into cubes

- 1 tbsp olive oil

- 1 onion (red or brown), finely chopped

- 2 cloves garlic, minced

- 1 red or green pepper, deseeded and chopped finely

- 100 g shiitake or chestnut mushrooms, finely sliced, or well minced if you have trouble swallowing (or you could use porcini mushrooms for a really earthy taste)

- 75 g shredded and finely chopped kale or similar dark green vegetable

- 2 heaped tsp dried mixed herbs (Provencal style is great)

- 4 eggs, beaten

- 250 ml skimmed milk

- 50 ml low-fat crème fraiche/sour cream

- 2 tbsps fresh chives, chopped (optional)

- salt and pepper, to taste

• 50 g strong cheddar cheese, shredded

Instructions

1. Spray or paint a one litre baking dish (approximately 27×18) with a little oil. Preheat the oven to 180C.

2. Pop the bread cubes into the oiled baking dish and set aside.

3. Heat the oil in a large frying pan.

4. Gently sauté the onions until soft, then add the remaining vegetables and the dried herbs.

5. Cook on a medium heat for about five minutes, until all are starting to soften.

6. Add a dash of stock or water to help the vegetables soften (although the mushroom and kale may release enough liquid).

7. Decant the cooked vegetables in to the baking dish. If you need to, whiz in a blender or food processor

8. In a medium mixing bowl whisk together the milk, crème fraiche, chives and the eggs, adding about 1 tsp of salt and a large pinch of pepper.

9. Pour this mixture over the vegetable topped bread cubes.

10. Gently press the mixture into the bread and allow to soak up for about five minutes.

11. Sprinkle over the cheese and bake in the preheated oven for about 25-30 minutes.

12. Allow to cool slightly before serving warm with a simple green salad or some cooked peas.

13. Pass the ketchup! Need more calories?

14. Add another tablespoon of oil, and use full-fat dairy.

15. Serves 2 generously.

Turkey Meatloaf

Preparation time

1 hour 12 minutes

Ingredients

- 1 tbsp olive oil or rapeseed oil

- 1 large onion, peeled and finely diced

- 2 cloves garlic, peeled and minced

- 2 medium carrots, peeled and finely diced

- 1 tbsp Worcestershire sauce

- 1 ½, tsp dried thyme

- 1 ½ tsp 'chicken seasoning' or 1 tsp salt and ½ tsp ground pepper

- 2 rounded tbsp tomato puree

- 500 g turkey mince

- 100 g porridge oats

- 2 eggs, beaten

- 60 ml vegetable or chicken stock

- 10 g parsley, chopped

- 100 ml tomato ketchup OR barbecue sauce

Instructions

1. In a frying pan, over a medium-hot heat, sauté the onions in the oil for about five minutes. Add the garlic and carrots to the pan and cook for a further eight minutes, or until the carrots begin to soften.

2. Add the next five ingredients and set aside to cool for a few minutes.

3. Blend the cooked vegetables if you are having trouble chewing.

4. Put the turkey mince and porridge oats into a large bowl and mix together.

5.   Add in the cooled vegetable mixture, beaten eggs, stock and parsley.

6. Mix well; it will look quite sloppy.

7.   Pat the meatloaf mixture into an oiled rectangular baking tin (approximately 28 x 18 cm) and cover with the ketchup or barbecue sauce. You can also form the mixture into a rectangular shape – about 10 cm/4 in high- on a well-oiled baking sheet. I tend to put it in the fridge for half an hour to firm up, but this is not necessary if you are putting the mix into a baking tin.

8. Bake at 170 C for 50 minutes to one hour, or until a meat thermometer registers 70C.

9. If you don't have a thermometer, ensure that the loaf is starting to pull away from the sides, or cut into the middle and see if steam escapes.

10. Serve 3-4 cm thick slices of the turkey meatloaf with mashed potato and celeriac, steamed dark greens (such as purple sprouting broccoli) and carrots, or red pepper strips.

Frittata, or Spanish Omelette

Preparation time

30 minutes

Ingredients

For one large skillet of frittata:

- 6 large organic eggs, well-beaten and seasoned with sea salt and freshly ground pepper

- a few glugs of olive oil (approx 2 tbsp)

- approx 2 sweet potatoes, boiled, and sliced (peeled if desired) to 1/2 cm or so

- 1 large Spanish or other mild onion (or two red onions), peeled and finely diced

- 1 large bag of fresh spinach, wilted, squeezed and chopped

- ½ tsp ground turmeric

- 1 tsp mustard seeds OR 1 tsp nigella seeds (optional)

- large nonstick frying pan

Ingredients

1. In the frying pan or cast iron skillet*, heat the oil over a medium to low heat.

2. Add onions and saute for a few minutes, then push aside and gently fry the sliced potatoes for a few minutes.

3. Spoon in your preferred seeds, if using.

4. Reorganise the onion and potatoes (i.e. even them out a bit).

5. Add the chopped spinach to the pan and beat the turmeric into the eggs.

6. If you have trouble chewing, perhaps breakdown the potatoes a bit with a fork and make sure your onions and spinach are well-chopped or blended.

7. Pour the seasoned eggs into the pan, making sure they are well-distributed.

8. Let mixture semi-set over a low heat. I usually cover the pan for most of the time.

9. Finish off under a hot grill or, if you are brave invert the frying pan onto a plate and slide the undercooked side back into the pan to finish. The undermost side will probably by quite golden brown with 'caught' oniony bits. This is the way it should be – you haven't burned it! If you have trouble chewing flip the frittata over before it gets brown and continue cooking until just cooked through.

10. Let it cool to almost room temperature (it doesn't taste nearly as nice straight from the

pan.). This also tastes fab cold and is perfect for picnics.

Melanzane Parmagiana (Aubergine Parmesan)

Prepartion time

1 hour

Ingredients

- Extra virgin olive oil

- 2 large aubergines/eggplants

- 125g baby spinach, wilted and squeezed dry (about ½ bag)

- Tomato Sauce (see below)

- 10g basil

- 1 ball fresh mozzarella, torn (lower fat is fine) OR full-fat ricotta

- 25 gm Parmesan cheese, freshly grated (optional)

- 25 gm fresh soft breadcrumbs (optional)

Instructions

1. Slick two baking trays with olive oil.

2. Slice the aubergines 1 cm thick and lay on the oiled trays.

3. Brush the aubergines with a little more oil.

4. Bake the aubergine at 200 C for about 20 minutes, or until very soft and looking golden brown.

5. Remove the aubergines from the oven.

6. For those with difficulty chewing perhaps remove the skin before slicing.

7. You could also shallow-fry these until golden, but use more oil.

8. Lower the oven temperature to 180 C. In a 8 by 12-inch pan (approximate size) place the largest slices in a single layer.

9. Top each with some sauce, a thin layer of spinach and some torn basil.

10. Continue layering up until all aubergines are used.

11. Top with last of the sauce, lay on the mozzarella or dollop on ricotta, sprinkle over the Parmesan and breadcrumbs.

12. Bake uncovered until the cheese melts and the crumbs are browned – about 25 minutes.

13. Sauce: 3 tbsp olive oil, 1 onion, diced, 2 cloves garlic, peeled and minced, 3 tbsp fresh thyme leaves or 1 tbsp dried, 1 medium carrot and 1 stalk celery – minced, 2 bay leaves, 2 x 454 gm tins best quality chopped tomatoes (Cirio are my favourite), salt to taste, sugar to taste (if tomatoes are a bit bitter).

14. Heat the oil in a medium heavy-bottomed pan (not aluminium).

15. Add the onion and sauté gently until onion is soft; add the garlic, thyme, carrot, bay and

celery and continue cooking for 15 minutes, until the carrot is quite soft.

16. Add the tomatoes with their juice and bring to the boil, stirring often.

17. Lower the heat and simmer for at least 30 minutes, until as thick as porridge;

18. season with salt, and maybe a pinch of sugar. Cool slightly, remove the bay leaves and whiz with a hand blender .You can keep

19. this sauce in the fridge for one week or freeze in an appropriate container for 3 months. Serves 4-6. This is also on the blog, from way back.

Steamed Fish with Puy Lentils and Salsa Verde

Prepartion time

30 minutes

Ingredients

- 200 g Puy lentils, washed and drained

- 1 bay leaf

- 1 small onion, peeled and halved

- salt and pepper

- 1 tbsp extra virgin olive oil

- 1 bunch of flat-leaf parsley (about 40 g)

- 6 basil leaves

- 20 mint leaves

- 1 small garlic clove, peeled

- 1 tbsp capers, rinsed and drained

- ½ tbsp Dijon mustard

- ½ tbsp fresh lemon juice

- 1 gherkin or 2 cornichon

- 3 tbsp extra virgin olive oil

- 2 anchovy fillets (optional but authentic)

- 4 x 150 g firm, white fish fillets

Instructions

1. Simmer the lentils, uncovered, with the bay leaf and onion in 500 ml of cold water for 20 minutes, or until the lentils are tender (have a nibble; they should taste 'done' but will look quite firm).

2. Drain, plucking out the bay leaf and onion.

3. Return the lentils to the pan and season.

4. Coat the lentils with the olive oil; cover and keep warm.

5. Mash the lentils with some of the cooking water and olive oil if you have trouble chewing and swallowing.

6. While the lentils are simmering, prepare the salsa. Some people pop everything into a food processor and blitz for a smooth sauce. Others mash everything with a pestle and mortar for a

more rustic dressing. Either is fine, although the latter is spectacularly messy if you are not practised. I tend to chop everything up on a board, scrape it into a mini food chopper and give it a quick pulse for a chunky, yet amalgamated texture. When serving this to children I also tend to add a teaspoon or two of water to the blending stage as this makes it less sharp.

7. Sort the fish just before serving. If you have a food steamer just place the fish on the perforated tray and steam for five minutes, or as recommended by the manufacturer. For those of you like me who have a less modern approach there are two recommended methods. If you have a pressure cooker use the trivet and basket that comes with it (but not locking the lid) and

steam the fish for five minutes over simmering water. Alternatively pour hot water in a large frying pan, place an upended heat-proof flat-bottomed ramekin (or similar) in the centre and top with a plate that accommodates the fish and fits, with a bit of steaming room, in the pan.

8.   Cover and steam for five minutes. If all that sounds a tremendous faff, poach in acidulated water (ie, add the juice of one lemon to enough lightly salted boiling water to just cover the fish) – turn off the heat when the water returns to the boil and leave for five minutes.

9. Drain and carry on with the dish.

10.   Regardless of the fish method used, place a generous spoonful of lentils on each plate, top

with a piece of fish and drizzle over some salsa.

Serve with lemon wedges. Serves 4

Pepper-Cheese Spread

 Prepartion time

25 minutes

Ingredients

- 100g roasted peppers in oil, drained

- 50 g sharp Cheddar cheese, shredded

- 50 g low fat soft cheese (or regular)

- 2 tbsp quality mayonnaise

- ¼ tsp garlic powder

- pinch of pepper

Instructions

1. Whizz everything up in a food processor and allow to 'come together' for 20 minutes before eating.

Creamy Polenta

Prepartion time

20 minutes

Ingredients

- 750 ml full-fat milk

- 1 small clove of garlic, lightly crushed and intact

- 1 small bay leaf

- salt and white pepper

- a pinch of nutmeg

- 75g quick cook polenta

- 100ml double cream/heavy cream/ crème fraiche

- 75g freshly grated Parmesan or Grana Padano cheese (NOT the stuff in a can!)

Instructions

1. Bring the milk to the boil and then add in the garlic, bay leaf, salt and pepper and nutmeg. Simmer for five minutes.

2. Use a slotted spoon to remove the bay leaf and garlic.

3. Slowly whisk in the polenta (pour it in in a steady stream, whisk all the time).

4. Cook the polenta on a low heat for 10 minutes, stirring so that it doesn't stick (which it really wants to do!).

5. Add in the cream and cheese, cooking for a further 2-3 minutes.

6. Eat warm with a big spoon.

Sardine Pate 'Provencale'

Prepartion time

 10 minutes

Ingredients

- 2 tins of natural sardine fillets – no brine or tomato sauce

- 125g soft cheese, light or full-fat according to need

- juice and zest of one small lemon

- small handful of parsley

- pinch of mixed herbs/herbes de Provence

* 10 green pitted olives

Instructions

1. Blend in a food processor until very smooth.

2. Have with bread, or even wrapped in soft lettuce leaves with some thin strips of cucumber.

3. Store in the refrigerator and use within three days.

Three-Fish Terrine

Prepartion time

30 minutes

Ingredients

- 100g salmon fillet
- 200g fresh haddock fillet (or similar)
- 100g undyed smoked haddock fillet (or similar)
- 100 ml double cream/heavy cream
- 2 large eggs, beaten
- salt and pepper
- mild paprika
- lemon juice plus lemon wedges

Instructions

1. Oil 4 ramekins and sprinkle very lightly with paprika.

2. Cut the salmon fillet into thin strips and divide between the ramekins, laying them neatly as this side will be uppermost when served.

3. Blend the smoked fish in a food processor

4. Add one-third of the beaten egg mixture and one-third of the cream, blending until smooth.

5. Set aside for now.

6. Blend together the fresh haddock and the remaining eggs and cream, adding a good pinch of salt and pepper, a teaspoon or so of lemon juice and a good pinch of paprika.

7. Put a tablespoon of the smoked fish mixture in each ramekin, then top with the fresh haddock mixture, press lightly to smooth.

8. Put the ramekins into a roasting tray; pour some boiling water into the tray so that it comes up about two-thirds the way, and bake in an oven preheated to 200C/400F for 30 minutes. OR microwave for eight minutes.

9. To serve, turn upside down on plate and garnish with soft lettuce (like salade mache) and a lemon wedge.

Miso-Glazed Fish

Preparation time

30 minutes

Ingredients

- 1 ½ tbsp brown sugar

- ½ tsp toasted sesame oil

- 1/4 tsp ground ginger

- 1 tbsp mirin, dry sherry or fresh lime juice

Instructions

1. Mix together the glaze ingredients until the brown sugar has completely dissolved.

2. Brush most of the glaze on both sides of the fish and leave to marinate for half an hour.

3. Preheat your grill/broiler and place the fish on a baking tray, then pop under the heat until the tops are starting to brown and the glaze

caramelizes – watch it to make sure it doesn't burn – about three minutes.

4. Take the fish from the grill/broiler, brush with the remaining glaze. Now either turn the heat to 180C/375C, or lightly cover the fish with foil (not touching the fish) and put on a lower rack, and cook until the fish is cooked through but still moist – about five minutes.

5. This glaze is also superb on baked aubergine/eggplant: slice an aubergine in half lengthways slash a diamond pattern into the flesh (not cutting the skin), oil and bake in a medium-hot oven for 20 minutes. Remove from the oven and spread over the miso glaze; place under a hot grill/broiler until bubbly.

6. Scoop out the tender flesh with a spoon and enjoy!

Pear and Cocoa Pudding

Prepartion time

45 minutes

- Ingredients

- 2 x 400g (approx weight) tins pear halves or quarters in juice

- 150g self-raising flour OR 150g plain flour + 1 tsp baking powder and ¼ tsp fine salt

- 25g cocoa powder

- 125g caster/fine sugar

• 150g butter or Earth Balance-type spread, plus extra for dish

• 2 medium eggs

• 2 tsp vanilla extract or ½ tsp vanilla paste/powder

Instructions

1. Drain the pears and lay in a pie dish or other ovenproof dish (e.g. 22cm square; I use an oval Le Creuset dish.

2. Pop the remaining ingredients in a food processor (or mix vigourously by hand) and whiz until it is completely smooth.

3. Drop spoonfuls of the batter over the pears and, with a wet spoon, carefully spread over the pears.

4. Bake in a 200C/400F oven for 25-30 minutes.

5. Allow to cool for a few minutes (if you can bear it!) before serving.

CURRIED CHICKEN SALAD

Prepartion time

10 minutes

Ingredients

• 2 small apples

• 1 rib celery

- 1/2 c mayonnaise

- 2 t curry powder or to taste

- 3 c diced cooked chicken

INSTRUCTIONS

1. Core the apples. Dice them and the celery small.

2. Put all ingredients in a large bowl.

3. Mix well.

4. Taste for seasoning.

5. Either serve at once, or chill and serve later - remembering that the curry will become more intense over time.

Salmon Quiche

Prepartion time

 Ingredients

• 1 9" prepared deep pie crust

• 10 oz Chicken of the Sea® Pink Salmon, Skinless & Boneless

• 1 tbsp dried bread crumbs, finely ground

• 1 tbsp parmesan cheese, grated

• 2 tsp olive oil

• 2/3 cup fresh red peppers, diced

• 1/3 cup fresh green onion, thin-sliced

• 1/2 tsp Old Bay® Seasoning

- 1/4 tsp hot sauce

- 2 tbsp reserved salmon liquid

- 6 fresh eggs

- 3/4 cup 2% milk

- 1 cup sharp cheddar cheese, shredded

- 1 tbsp fresh parsley, minced

Instructions

1. Prick pie crust with fork and bake at 425°F for 7 minutes or until lightly browned.

2. Drain salmon and reserve liquid. Chop salmon, toss with bread crumbs and Parmesan.

3. Heat olive oil in a sauté pan, medium heat. Add peppers and onions.

4. Cook until onions are translucent. Add Old Bay Seasoning and hot sauce; toss with reserved salmon liquid.

5. Simmer until liquid is reduced by 90%.

6. Blend eggs and milk. Add cheese and parsley to the egg mixture.

7. Blend in cooked vegetables and salmon/bread crumb mixture.

8. Pour into pie crust and place in 350°F oven for 35 minutes or until done.

CREAMY CHICKEN CASSEROLE WITH BUTTERNUT SQUASH & APPLES

Prepartion time

30 minutes

Ingredients

- 1 pound ground chicken

- 1 can low-fat Cream of Chicken Soup

- 1/2 cup low-fat milk

- 1 apple peeled and diced

- 1 cup frozen butternut squash

- 1/2 cup shredded cheddar cheese

- 1/2 cup whole wheat panko breadcrumbs

Instructions

1. Preheat oven to 350 degrees F.

2. In a saute pan cook ground chicken until cooked through.

3. Pour cream of chicken soup and milk into ground chicken and mix to combine.

4. Heat chicken over medium until sauce begins to bubble.

5. Add diced apple and butternut squash.

6. Cook for 10-15 minutes or until apples soften.

7. Pour creamy chicken into a baking dish.

8. Spread 1/2 cup of shredded cheddar cheese on top of the casserole.

9. Top with 1/2 cup of whole wheat panko breadcrumbs.

10. Bake for 10 minutes or until cheese is melted.

Creamy Carrot Cauliflower Soup

Prepartion time

35 minutes

Ingredients

- 1 Tablespoon butter or olive oil

- 1 large onion, peeled & chopped

- 3 – 5 cloves garlic, peeled & chopped

- 1 cup chopped carrots

- 1/2 of a large head of cauliflower, broken into florets

- 2 cups water

- 2 teaspoons better than boullion (chicken or vegetable)

- 1 bay leaf

- About 1 cup (2 oz.) shredded MontAmore cheese (or other flavorful cheese)

- 4 oz. Greek cream cheese (or Neufchatel)

- 1 cup 1% milk

For garnish:

- Extra shredded cheese (or carrots)

- Fresh thyme sprigs

Instructions

1. Heat a soup pot over medium heat, then add the butter or olive oil. Add the onion and garlic and cook until the onion is very soft and translucent, about 10 minutes.

2. Add the carrot and cook a few minutes longer, then add the cauliflower, water, boullion and bay leaf. Cover and cook for about 10 – 15 minutes or until the cauliflower is nice and tender.

3. Remove the bay leaf and pour the rest into a blender. Add the shredded cheese, Greek cream cheese and milk and blend until smooth.

4. Serve hot, garnished with shredded carrot or shredded cheese and fresh thyme.

Beef and Bean Enchilada Casserole

Prepartion time

40 minutes

Ingredients

* 8 ounces lean ground beef

* 1/2 cup chopped sweet onion

* 1 teaspoon chili powder

* 1/2 teaspoon ground cumin

- One 15-ounce can pinto beans, drained and rinsed

- One 4-ounce can diced green chiles

- 8 ounces sour cream (light is fine)

- 2 tablespoons all-purpose flour

- 1/4 teaspoon garlic powder

- Eight 6-inch corn tortillas

- 1½ cups enchilada sauce

- 1½ to 2 cups mixed cheddar/Jack shredded cheese

topping suggestions:
 chopped tomatoes, sour cream, guacamole

Prepartion time

1. Preheat the oven to 350 degrees F. Spray a 9x13-inch pan or 2-quart baking dish with nonstick spray.

2. In a large skillet, cook the ground beef and onion together over medium heat until the beef is browned and the onion is tender.

3. Drain any fat, if needed.

4. Stir in the chili powder, cumin, beans, and chiles; set aside.

5. In a medium bowl, whisk together the sour cream, flour and garlic powder.

High Protein Tuna Salad

Prepartion time

10 minutes

INGREDIENTS

• 1 can tuna packed in water, drained

• 1 egg, hardboiled

• 2 tbsp plain Greek yogurt

• Spices and vegetables of your choice, based on

tolerance

INSTRUCTIONS

1.   Drain the tuna well and pour into medium-sized mixing bowl

2. Cut the egg into bite-sized pieces and place into bowl

3. Add Greek yogurt, spices, and vegetables based on your tolerance

4. Mix well.

5.   Add more Greek yogurt if it isn't moist enough

6. Eat straight from the bowl, or spread on a thin cracker to eat.

Easy Pureed Vegetable Soup

Prepartion time

50 minutes

Ingredients

- 2 tablespoons extra virgin olive oil, such as Kirkland's

- OPTIONAL: 1 teaspoon anchovy paste

- 2 cups chopped Spanish onion

- 1 leek, halved lengthwise and sliced 1/2-inch thick

- 2 carrots, peeled and chopped

- 1 red bell pepper, seeded and chopped

- 3 celery stalks, chopped

- 10 cloves garlic, chopped

- 1/2 teaspoon Himalayan salt, plus more as desired

- 1/8 teaspoon ground pepper

- 1 teaspoon Italian seasoning

- 8 cups vegetable broth

- 2 cups cauliflower florets

- 2 – 14.5 ounce cans diced tomatoes, drained

- OPTIONAL: 5 large handful baby spinach

- Juice from 1 whole lemon

- 1 – 15 ounce can garbanzo beans, rinsed and drained

Instructions

1. Heat the oil and anchovy paste (if using) in a large heavy stockpot over medium heat. Add the onion and leeks, and cook, stirring occasionally, until translucent, about 8-minutes.

2. Add the carrots, bell pepper, celery, garlic, salt, pepper and Italian seasoning. Cook for 5 minutes, stirring occasionally.

3. Pour in the vegetable broth, cover the pot, and bring to a boil.

4. Add the cauliflower and tomatoes, lower heat and simmer for 10 minutes, or until cauliflower softens.

5. Add the spinach (if using) and lemon juice and cook for a further 30 seconds, then remove from the heat.

6. Taste and adjust seasoning, if necessary.

7. Use a hand stick blender, such as Cuisinart's Smart Stick to process until smooth and creamy. (See notes below if you do not have a handheld stick blender.) Add garbanzo beans (if using) and puree again.

8. Serve warm.

CREAMY CHICKEN

Prepartion time

10 minutes

Ingredients

- 4 cups chicken breasts, cooked

- 1/3 cup (112 g) mayonnaise

- 1 cup (101 g) Celery, thinly sliced

- 1/4 cup (35.75 g) Almonds, sliced

- 1 teaspoon (1 teaspoon) Kosher Salt

- 1-2 teaspoons (1 teaspoons) ground black pepper

Instructions

1. Place cooked chicken meat in your Kitchenaid or other stand mixer. Use the paddle to shred the chicken. Do not skip this step! This is the key to why this salad is very creamy, moist, and just delicious. You can do this by pulsing in a food processor as well. This step is critical to finely shredding the chicken

2. Mix in everything into the chicken, and eat.

EASY & MOIST STRAWBERRY BREAD

Prepartion time

50 minutes

Ingredients

• 2 eggs, at room temperature

• 1/2 cup (100 grams) regular sugar or unrefined cane sugar (see notes)

• 1/2 scant cup (80-90 grams) vegetable oil (I used expeller-pressed canola oil)

• 1 cup (250 grams) Plain or Greek-style yogurt (see notes)

• 1 tsp vanilla extract

- 1 ½ cup + 1Tbsp (200 grams) all-purpose flour or white spelt flour

- 1 ½ tsp baking powder

- 1/8 tsp fine salt

- 1 ½ cup (approx 200 grams) strawberries, diced

JAM GLAZE

- 3 Tbsp Strawberry or apricot jam

Instructions

1. Preheat the oven to 350°F/180°C degrees and place the rack in the middle position.

2. Grease a 9x5x2.5 inch loaf pan with butter or simply line the pan with parchment paper.

3. In a bowl, beat eggs and sugar with a fork or a whisk.

4. Then add oil, yogurt (not cold), vanilla essence, and whisk to a smooth consistency.

5. In a second bowl, whisk flour, baking powder, and salt.

6. Add the dry ingredients to the wet ingredients, stir with a spatula until just combined.

7. Do not overmix.

8. Fold the diced strawberries gently into the batter, using a spatula and trying to distribute them evenly.

9. Scrape the batter into the prepared loaf pan and smooth the top. Bake for about 40-45 minutes, until a skewer inserted into the center of the cake comes out clean.

10. When the cake is done, remove it from the oven and place on a wire rack to cool. You can serve it plain or glazed with jam. I

11. glazed it brushing some warm strawberry jam on top (see notes)*. Enjoy!

Creamy Mashed Potatoes

Prepartion time

45 minutes

Ingredients

Steaming the Potatoes

- • 1 1/2 to 2 lb large red potatoes

- • 1 tsp sea salt

- • bay leaves (optional)

Mashing the Potatoes

- • 6 tbsp non-dairy milk

- • 1 to 2 tbsp non-dairy butter or oil

- • sea salt, to taste

- • white pepper, to taste

Instructions

Steaming the Potatoes

1. To start, gather a pot and steaming basket. Add about one inch of water to the pot and bring to a boil.

2. In the meantime, peel and cut the potatoes in half or into even-sized, large chunks.

3. Once the water comes to a boil, place the potatoes into the steamer basket and place into the pot. If using bay leaves, place them on top of the potatoes. Sprinkle the potatoes with the salt and cover.

4. Turn the heat to medium and let steam until a knife inserted into the thickest part goes in with ease, about 20 to 30 minutes. The potatoes must be fully cooked or else you will have lumpy potatoes.

5. To start, gather a pot and steaming basket.

6. Add about one inch of water to the pot and bring to a boil.

7. In the meantime, peel and cut the potatoes in half or into even-sized, large chunks.

8. Once the water comes to a boil, place the potatoes into the steamer basket and place into the pot. If using bay leaves, place them on top of the potatoes. Sprinkle the potatoes with the salt and cover.

9. Turn the heat to medium and let steam until a knife inserted into the thickest part goes in with ease, about 20 to 30 minutes. The potatoes must be fully cooked or else you will have lumpy potatoes.

Note: You can substitute russets; however, they will not provide the same creamy texture. Yukon Gold potatoes can also be used with good results.

Drying the Potatoes

1. Once the potatoes are done, remove the steamer basket and drain the water from the pot. Place the potatoes into the pot.

2. Cover the surface of the potatoes with a clean kitchen cloth for a few minutes.

3. This will help to absorb any excess moisture.

Matshing me

1. To mash the potatoes, use an electric hand mixer on low speed to first break up the large chunks of potato.

2. Then add the non-diary milk and butter and whip the potatoes on high speed until smooth and creamy.

3. Taste for seasoning and serve immediately.